THE WTF DIVORCE JOURNAL

THE RAW, THE REAL, AND THE RIDICULOUSLY RELATABLE

WTF DIVORCE
The Journal

To my kids, Cameron, Brooks, and Remy.
You motivate me to take chances
and do big things. I'm proud to be your Dad,
and watch the people you're becoming.
-Rob

Kennedy and Cade, my reason for trying to
be a little bit better each day.
-Kristy

ADVANCE PRAISE

"WTF Divorce is our daily dose of laughter - a divorce therapist in memes and a vulnerable haven for divorced women & men."
-Monika Casey & Tom Arnold
Divorce Party Podcast

"Love WTF Divorce! The content is funny, insightful, and helps you get through the hard days of divorce."
- Alessandra Martinet, @mamasguidetodivorce

"WTF Divorce is an innovative, supportive community that will make you laugh, feel connected, and help you navigate divorce."
-Meagan Norris, @meagannorriscoaching

"WTF Divorce offers you humor, knowledge, and community. The key ingredients for surviving a sh*tstorm."
-Andrea Rappaport, @theandrearappaport
How Not To Suck At Divorce Podcast

WHAT PEOPLE ARE SAYING

Thank you for doing what you do 😉 it's nice sharing this roller coaster pad

This is THERAPY

Completely. Your account has helped me so much

As someone who is scared to death to even contemplate a divorce from a toxic, narcissistic husband, your page has been a godsend!

Im soooo happy I found your account some times I felt so lonely with what I was going through

Thanks for this Instagram page. It's helped me seeing other people dealing with the same pain.

Welcome, I wouldn't wish divorce in my worst enemy. It hurts like hell and for my case never ending. This page has made me feel less alone.

Yes! Thank you! And thank you for having a page that makes us all Feel less alone 🖤

That really hit home! So glad I just found your profile - LOVE it 👏👏 thank you for creating this every day

Some of these posts are so relatable and so real . Divorce certainly is one of those things that you picture as the end of your problems and is just - 🤯

I could relate to so many of those comments. It's such a hard thing to overcome and not lose yourself but also create a better person.

Thank you for sharing that. Hopefully hearing from others helps us all feel like we're not the only ones.

I thinks it powerful to hear from others ,It makes you feel ok about your own situation . Thank you for all the work you do on here 🙏💪 🖤

You're page is amazing! Has got me through some hard times! 🖤

All great advice!
Love what you are doing with this account, it's been a tremendous help, thank you!

Just found your acct. I'll follow once the ink is dry on the divorce papers. I know you get lots of "thank you for what you're doing," but here's another one — thank you.

This feed is hilarious, heartwarming, healing and tender. Great job!

I feel seen! THIS! This post means it happens to others — NOT just me. Thank you.

Thaaannnkkk youuuuuu for being so fucking relatable..🥲🥲🥲

Just wanted to say I really love this account. It's helping me a lot in my healing journey. You're doing good work.

And this happened too 🤦‍♀️. It's amazing you feel so alone and then you read others experiences. Thanks for bringing people together 🙏

OMG, thank you so much for posting this! Now I can read it and laugh, instead of feel sad!!

JUST FOR THE RECORD DARLING,

NOT ALL POSITIVE CHANGES FEEL POSITIVE IN THE BEGINNING.

-S.C. LOURIE

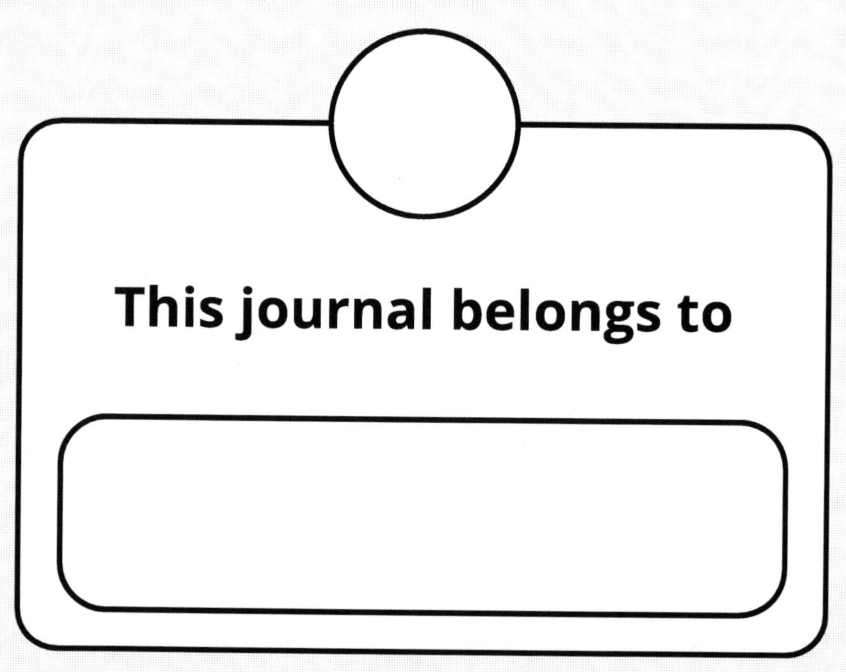

And I’ll say what I want :)

INTRODUCTION

Divorce...WTF, right?

Even though statistics show that 50% of marriages end in divorce, most days it feels like you're the only one going through it.

Your married friends don't get it.
Your family doesn't get it.
Your ex...they never got it.

At WTF Divorce, we get it.

We have always described WTF Divorce as the best friend who hosted the party, and YOU'RE invited.

We are here to encourage you to cuss, yell, make bad decisions, and feel the full spectrum of emotions that come with divorce.

Want to burn your wedding album?
We will send the matches.

Want to anonymously mail a bag of d*cks to your ex?
Put our return address.

Want to date 4 different people in one weekend?
We'll set it up.

We are here to meet you where you're at.

If you are over buying journals and never getting past page 5 of gratitude lists, and are ready to lean into the ugly, the petty, and the necessary emotions.

This journal is for you.

Our 117,000 IG followers have opened up and shared their struggles with divorce, co-parenting, and dating again.

Filled with inspiring quotes, laugh-out-loud memes, real journal samples and

Questions like:

- What's 1 thing you'd have told yourself before you got married?
- What's the most annoying divorce advice you received?
- What's 1 relationship truth you learned from your divorce?

It's quick. It's dirty. It's fun. It's WTF Divorce.

And you're invited to join us.

Oh, but first - I almost forgot - you've also got some **FREE bonuses** to look forward to.

If you want to get a head start, you can access everything by going to:

www.WTFdivorce.com/journal

If you find this book helpful, **please leave a quick review** on Amazon, and tell your friends about it.

This helps it find its way to those who need it, and it would really mean a lot to us.

Thank you.
-Rob & Kristy

HOW TO USE THIS JOURNAL

Welcome to the WTF Divorce journal.

A place where we are sharing with you some of the best things our friends have told us while they've been at the party.

It also includes places for you to dabble, dream and digest the feelings you have as you navigate and reflect on this stage of life.

It is not meant to be homework.

Nor does it need to be completed in its entirety.

Each mini-section includes a journaling prompt, follower responses, a raw quote,
a snarky meme, and an affirmation.

See which sections, topics or prompts speak to you.

Pay attention to the ones that make you nervous....and dive in!

I am healing everyday

Rewrite the affirmation

A LETTER TO MYSELF POST-DIVORCE

@WTFdivorce

WELCOME TO THE NEXT CHAPTER OF YOUR LIFE.

EVERYTHING THAT HAS HAPPENED IS JUST A PART OF YOUR STORY.

THERE ARE PARTS THAT WERE SAD,

PARTS THAT WERE BEAUTIFUL,

PARTS THAT WERE UGLY,

AND PARTS THAT YOU THOUGHT WOULD BREAK YOU.

HERE'S THE GOOD NEWS.

THE STORY ISN'T OVER AND YOU WERE ALWAYS THE WRITER.

KEEP TURNING THE PAGES.

EVERY CHOICE AND EVERY STEP TOOK YOU HERE, SO DON'T BE MAD AT THE PAST.

GREAT LOVE IS REAL.

**YOU DESERVE IT.
YOUR KIDS
DESERVE TO SEE IT.**

AND IT CAN STILL BE A PART OF YOUR FUTURE.

WRITE YOURSELF A SHORT LETTER

WTF

I forgive myself

Rewrite the affirmation

When did you know it was time to get divorced?

Write your answer in the box above
Follower Responses (Circle Ones You Connect With)

when i dreaded opening the door	when i realized that my life was easier when he was traveling and not around	when i stoped hoping for change
when he cheated, emotionally and physically	when she lied to me about where she was and wouldn't answer her phone.	when I did not want my kids to see anymore, how bad he was treating me
when he touched me and i cringed. i flet violated	when I realized his work was more important than my health	the day before the wedding
I knew it was time when my son said he did not like the way dad spoke to me.	when he implied we were both narcissists	soooo many of these answers ring true for me!!!!

When did you know it was time to get divorced?

When I didn't have the energy to fight for it anymore

THE ONLY TIME WE GET OFF THE FENCE ABOUT LEAVING A RELATIONSHIP IS WHEN ONE THING HAPPENS:

WHEN THE PAIN OF STAYING WITH THIS PERSON BECOMES GREATER THAN THE PAIN OF LEAVING THEM.

-CINDY STIBBARD
@cindy.stibbard

Falling in love makes you do stupid things.

One time I even got married.

-ALESSANDRA MARTINET
@mamasguidetodivorce

You got this

Rewrite the affirmation

What's the #1 reason you got divorced?

Write your answer in the box above
Follower Responses (Circle Ones You Connect With)

Lord, there isn't enough room to answer that	Lack of respect	I knew I derserved better
Cheating, lies	Partner is underfunctioning with covered narcissistic behaviors	He could not make a decision and i was tired of doing it all.
Walked in on her naked with another man and she gaslit the hell out of me over it	my health issues were too hard on him	his alcoholism led to my affair. we could not recover.
Stopped showing up for each other	he had a baby with another women, and hid it 2 yrs, she made him confess	isolating me from friends and family

What's the #1 reason you got divorced?

Did not want my kids to think that was an ok way for their mom to be treated

DID HE LIE TO YOU ABOUT WHO HE WAS?

OR DID YOU LIE TO YOURSELF ABOUT WHO HE WAS?

-UNKNOWN

What's 1 thing you'd have told yourself before you got married?

Write your answer in the box above

Follower Responses (Circle Ones You Connect With)

Break up with him! these things that bother you now are all big things	**Marriage is not the goal. A loving, healthy, safe relationship is the goal.**	**Trust your instincts oops**
You are not obliged	**Make sure you love yourself first. That will show how others should love you.**	**Date longer. Discuss LT life goals to make sure you're on same page beyond 1st few yrs**
He will turn into his father!	**Mom knows best**	**It's not that bad to end up alone or marry later**
It's okay to back out now. you will be lose everything if it goes south later	**Don't take everything so personally. What others do is about themselves.**	**You know better.**

What's 1 thing you'd have told yourself before you got married?

Wait and listen to that still small voice that was really the truth!

Now that you're getting divorced, can I get a refund for your 3-day destination wedding?

-UNKNOWN

F This

LEAVING AN UNHEALTHY RELATIONSHIP WILL LITERALLY CHANGE THE COURSE OF YOUR ENTIRE LIFE.

IF THAT'S THE BRAVEST THING YOU EVER DO, IT'S ENOUGH.

-MICHELLE DEMPSEY
@themichelledempsey

I'm ok with being on my own

Rewrite the affirmation

SOMETIMES WHEN THINGS ARE FALLING APART,

THEY MAY ACTUALLY BE FALLING INTO PLACE

-BARBARA MEZEI
@joyfulsmolthings

What was 'the divorce talk' like for you?

Write your answer in the box above

Follower Responses (Circle Ones You Connect With)

He had been pretending, and in one night knocked my reality and future upside down.	No talk. He came home while I was at work and took things. I thought we were robbed for a minute.	it was super uncomfotrable, but I did it.
Found out he hadn't been monogamous since year 2 to 18 and lied about his needs	He went to store for dog food and I sent him an email with all the details.	told him & said he'd move after the holidays but changed his mind and didn't tell me.
mortgage renewal - Him: "what should we do" Me: " sell house & divorce"	"I'm filing."	Talk? I had to flee with my son
4th (maybe more honestly) affair partner in 2 years finally told me what was going on	had the talk again but he wouldn't leave. 5 years later, he's been out since Jan!	Me telling him to go after making him log n2 his secret email acct & reading notes

What was 'the divorce talk' like for you?

Less scary than the anticipation of it

**“I WASTED A LOT OF ENERGY
OVER THE YEARS
STAYING IN SPACES
WHERE I THOUGHT,**

**‘IF I COULD JUST SHOW TO
THIS PERSON MY LIGHT,
AND MY HEART,
AND VALUE, THEY'D
RECIPROCATE THE ENERGY.**

**LESSON: YOUR WORTH IS
NOT PREDICATED ON
WHETHER OR NOT OTHERS
CAN RECOGNIZE IT IN YOU.”**

-Joél Leon
@JoelakaMaG

A marriage license should expire every 4 years so you can decide if you even wanna renew that mf

@wordgasm

Would you have renewed at year 4? How about year 8?

I will be ok.

Rewrite the affirmation

What's one of your favorite breakup songs?

Write your answer in the box above

Follower Responses (Circle Ones You Connect With)

Lose you to love me	Firework	I will survive. The ex despises this song so it even more fitting
IDGAF	Cardigan	Blink 182 don't leave me
Not my X but my Y	irreplaceable	Free Falling Tom Petty
Highway to hell	Unstoppable	Flowers

What's one of your favorite breakup songs?

ABCDEFU was my anthem at the beginning

"MY BIGGEST FEAR IS THAT MY CHILDREN WON'T KNOW WHAT A HEALTHY RELATIONSHIP LOOKS LIKE.

BUT MY BIGGEST SOURCE OF PRIDE IS THAT THEY WILL KNOW HOW TO FIND HAPPINESS ON THEIR OWN."

-KRISTY TIESING
@kristy_anne2_

My ex is somewhere telling his new girlfriend how bad I was, and she's smiling and thinking she's made it in life.

Two idiots.

-Unknown

WTF

I trust in myself

Rewrite the affirmation

How did you let people know you were divorced?

I need ideas - I was married for 25 years....	Deleted all of his pics and changed my profile pic	My ex posted a pic of himself crying and told all of FB
Changed my profile to my maiden name	Christmas card of just the kids and myself	Never on social media. Only called close friends
Not me, but my ex immediately changed his Facebook status	getting my doctorate + name change, announced myself as the future Dr. Maiden name	She didn't tell anyone. I told people when I absolutely had to.
changed my relationship status to single	My gf and I were just trying to come up with a clever way to do this	I turned our wedding website into a divorce announcement, shared on FB

How did you let people know you were divorced?

Invited allll my friends and fam to my divorce party...it took a long time and needed celebrating

When the wife starts posting selfies and the husband changes his profile pic to the kids

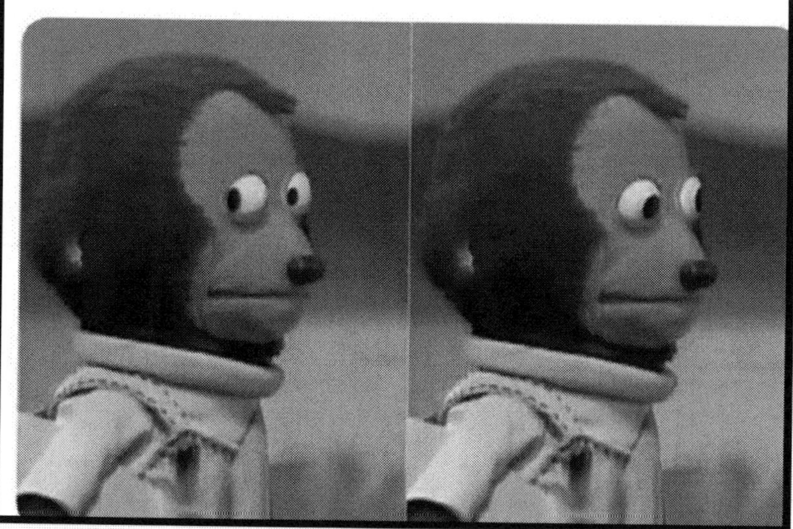

What's a sign of divorce on social media?

- Wife posting thirst traps
- Inspirational quotes galore
- ______________________________

"I AM NOT GOING TO LIVE MY LIFE BECAUSE OF SOMETHING SOMEONE MIGHT SAY."

-CHRISTINA AGUILERA
@xtina

Life has a different plan for me

Rewrite the affirmation

How much did your divorce cost?

Write your answer in the box above
Follower Responses (Circle Ones You Connect With)

Triple digits	**Not divorced 21k so far**	**6k**
Over $15,000 so far and no end in sight.	**12k still going**	**$948 - it's easier when they give up because they know you're the better arguer**
Still paying.... still going	**50k**	**$10,000... looking at an additional $20,000 if it has to go to trial**
15k legal fees. A lot more in losing the house though	**$30k and still not done**	**So far $60,000 and not even to mediation yet**

How much did your divorce cost?

0-$5,000

$5,000-$15,000

$15,000+

DO YOU KNOW WHY DIVORCE IS SO EXPENSIVE?

BECAUSE IT'S WORTH IT.

-MILLIONS OF EX-HUSBANDS AND EX-WIVES

Happiness is inside me

Rewrite the affirmation

What's 1 thing you'd tell someone to include in their divorce settlement?

Write your answer in the box above

Follower Responses (Circle Ones You Connect With)

Schedule around Christmas!	**Specific time exchanges (reg schedule & holidays), including transportation**
Sleepovers with a new partner and the kids. College funds. Therapy costs for kids.	**Right of first refusal**
How long til his new gf can move in with our kids?!?	**Cell phone bills and car insurance for the children. Got stuck with both of those.**
If your college kids have a car. Who will pay for insurance, repairs etc & phones.	**How you're handling medical expenses**

What's 1 thing you'd tell someone to include in their divorce settlement?

Don’t rely on advice from your family. They don’t get it.

YOU DIDN'T BECOME SELFISH.

YOU BECAME HARDER TO MANIPULATE.

DON'T CONFUSE THE TWO.

-UNKNOWN

If you listen closely, you can hear the sound of your ex's new flame realizing that you weren't the crazy one.

-ANDREA RAPPAPORT
@theandrearappaport

THEIR REACTION TO YOU HOLDING THEM ACCOUNTABLE, IS NOT YOUR BURDEN TO CARRY.

-TRACY MOORE-GRANT
@amicabledivorcenetwork

I forive myself for past relationships

Rewrite the affirmation

Did your church/temple support you in your divorce?

Nope. Nada.	Divorce Care group was amazing. Find one near you.	Most did
I felt ostracized	I moved home (3 states away). Our church family abandoned me. My new church family suported me.	hahahaha "church" is the least Christian thing I know
Some did, some did not. Not who I expected	Yeah they really stepped up and kept checking in	We left it and found another supportive school community
No	Took a few years but made some really great single mom connections at the masjid	No, sons's catholic school said we were from a broken family

Did your church/temple support you in your divorce?

The Church was very pleased with my decisions, being I divorced the devil

"YOU CAN CHOOSE TO LET ADVERSITY FUEL PAIN AND POWERLESSNESS,

OR YOU CAN CHOOSE TO LET IT FUEL GRIT AND DETERMINATION."

-MEAGAN NORRIS
@meagannorriscoaching

I thought I'd never have good sex again... but then I got divorced!

-SADIE MARIE
@sadiesdivorcedandhappy

WTF

IF CHANGING YOUR LIFE SITUATION WAS EASY,

YOU'D HAVE DONE IT YEARS AGO.

-HEIDI BROCKE
@coachingwithdrheidi

I will no longer be taken for granted

Rewrite the affirmation

Did you have religious issues with your co-parent?

My ex became a Jehovah witness.. all because he wanted to date one. AWFUL

Said no way once we were divorced

My ex told me God told him to get a divorce

Ex is heavy Catholic and I'm open. He wants our son to be Catholic but I want him to be open.

Ex doesn't believe in evolution. "No way we came from monkeys!"

It's all on me to keep it going.

Wants our kid to go to religious private school with his step kids. Neither of us is religious

Ex is religious. I don't want to raise children w/ differetn values. I feel controlled.

My 5yo daughter mentioned god once and my ex blamed me for it.

He's atheist. I'm not. We agreed to raise in my faith until kids were older to choose.

Wants our kids to be baptized and go on missions for LDS church. They don't want to.

Son and daughter baptized without my knowledge or consent.

Did you have religious issues with your co-parent?

Ex uses religion as a facade in front of others. She thinks it makes me look bad I'm agnostic.

"I HAD BUILT MY LIFE ON TRYING TO BE ALL THINGS TO ALL PEOPLE, AND I JUST COULDN'T DO IT ANYMORE."

-GWYNETH PALTROW
@gwynethpaltrow

I will get through this

Rewrite the affirmation

How did your employer support you during divorce?

by being understanding & supportive, taking things off my plate or giving me more time	firing me hahaha	understanding, but more workload, needed the distraction
none what so ever	my boss listens to what i need	supportive in every step of the way. encouraged to take days off when needed
allowed me to come into work late	what support?	by riding me about everything and trying to fire me
gave me increased flexibility for mental health time	they let me take time off.	supportive in every step of the way. encouragement take time off when needed

How did your employer support you during divorce?

Told her I decided to divorce. She handed me a tissue, said 'I'll be fine, it's his loss.' I got a promotion too!

DELETE THE OLD VERSION OF ME IN YOUR HEAD.

IT EXPIRED.

-UNKNOWN

Signing my divorce papers was the first time I ever ‘finished’ with my ex.

@WTFdivorce

Keep going

Rewrite the affirmation

What happened to your pets in the divorce?

Write your answer in the box above

Follower Responses (Circle Ones You Connect With)

I kept my cats and now new bf has won their approval	He kept the cat. Didn't have any other pets.	I saved him from my careless ex. Couldn't even keep a dog healthy
I got the dog as I had the better financial ability and supportive family to help care for him.	Dogs go with the kids. 50/50 custody. It was the one request our kids had	He wouldn't even try to listen or compromise. He claimed her and refuses to let me see her or share.
Took mine	I got them both!!!	She stole our dog
I kept them. He didn't even want them after 6 years. I'm so glad I don't have to share them.	We share 'custody' of our dog. i hate it as it's a link to him but I rely on his help to look after the dog	He adopted 2 dogs 3 m bef leaving home. then said he knew wated to leave 2 y bef. And left me the dogs.

What happened to your pets in the divorce?

She kept the dog, I got a new one.

"I KNOW REGRETS CAN BE CATALYSTS FOR GOOD THINGS.

NOT TO TALK LIKE A HALLMARK CARD, BUT IT'S TRUE."

-JAMES MARSDEN
@james_marsden

I am a good person

Rewrite the affirmation

How long did your ex's relationship with their affair partner last?

Audience Responses (circle ones that resonate):

Still going	Please post the answers	Refuses to answer this question :(
Married Now	Still Going - post divorce 1.5 years	Well they have an oops baby and thus, got married. Just call me Reba
Almost 3years	1 year and he cheated on her too.	Ended before we did
5 years	They are married now. And I feel sorry for him...	Going on 4 years...

How long did your ex's relationship with their affair partner last?

1 year and he cheated on her too.

Write an embarrassing secret you kept about them that you want to tell everyone:

....

....

....

....

WTF

YOU WEREN'T ASKING FOR TOO MUCH,

YOU WERE JUST ASKING THE WRONG PERSON.

-SABRINA ZOHAR
@do.the.work.podcast

When an anniversary post says, "We've had our ups and downs" that means he cheated.

-Unknown

SOMETIMES THE ONLY CLOSURE YOU NEED

IS UNDERSTANDING YOU DESERVE BETTER

-BRADLEY RICHARDSON
@imbradleyrichardson

Fuck this shit

Rewrite the affirmation

What's the most annoying divorce advice you received?

Write your answer in the box above

Follower Responses (Circle Ones You Connect With)

What happend to him? he was such a great guy!	We always thought he was awkward anyways.	You are so lucky to be able to sleep someone new.
You can forgive his cheating if you try	You should have waited	"You need to start dating right now" Made me sick to think about.
Was it really that bad that you ahd to leave? He's such a great guy	Tell her to #*}% off (we have two kids)	After he left, I got told "You should read the power of the praying wife"
"He should not get to see his son since he has not paid" ... and let that be used against me?	"You will meet someone" No.	But he was your husband, so you really can't call that 'sexual assault'.

What's the most annoying divorce advice you received?

We always thought he was awkward anyways.

I HATE WHEN PEOPLE REFER TO SINGLE PARENTS AS HAVING A "BROKEN HOME".

IT'S NOT.

YOU KNOW WHAT'S A BROKEN HOME?

HAVING A HOUSE FULL OF PEOPLE WHO SHOULDN'T BE TOGETHER AND BLEED THAT TOXIC ENERGY INTO THEIR KIDS.

THAT IS A BROKEN HOME.

-ALESSANDRA MARTINET
@mamasguidetodivorce

If you are sad, just remember there's someone meeting your ex and thinking they found true love.

-Unknown

I am free to build a life I want

Rewrite the affirmation

MAYBE YOU DON'T NEED MORE SELF-HELP TIPS OR INSPIRATIONAL QUOTES.

MAYBE YOU NEED MORE LAUGHTER AND POSITIVE EXPERIENCES WITH SAFE PEOPLE.

-JACQUELYN TENAGLIA
@no.bs.therapist

I am not broken

Rewrite the affirmation

What's some terrible support that you got after divorce?

None. People avoid you like you have a virus.	Lol we tried talking him out of it lol ummm no	I never liked him anyways
My mom kept inviting my ex to dinner "but he's always been at dinners with us"	People telling me to look the other way on infidelity "to keep fam together" Forget happiness	Aren't you worried about the kids?
Parents told me I was hurting my daughter by leaving and should stay.	Our couples therapist said she knew we'd get a divorce after appt#2.	Some people telling me "not to worry I'll find a man soon". Like really?! That's the last thing.
"What a shame, there isn't a way you two can work it out?"	From familly, "have you really thoughts this through"? Umm train is leaving get on board.	My friends kept praying my marraige would be healed. My ex was verbally abusive

What's some terrible support that you got after divorce?

'I would have left after the first time!' Yeah ok thanks!

**"PEOPLE SAY,
'OH, GOD, HOW DEVASTATING TO GO THROUGH A DIVORCE.'**

DID I WISH FOR THIS TO HAPPEN TO MY FAMILY?

NO.

BUT EVERYONE IS HEALTHY;

WE'RE MOVING ON WITH OUR LIVES."

-HEIDI KLUM

Some relationships truly inspire me to be single.

-Unknown

This shit is hard sometimes

Rewrite the affirmation

What did you do with your wedding album?

Threw it out.	Threw in the trash, wedding dress too	Hidden at the top of my closet.
I still have it. It's empty actually. After 9 years, the photographer did not give us the pics	Last day of the 6 month waiting period & burned all the pictures into the pit	never developed them. some of his fam brought their black clouds
Thankfully never paid thousands to make one!!	Gave them to my ex to decide what to do with it	Never got one... just this big framed photo in the living room that is ripped apart
Nothing yet... I'd probably just tear out the pages	Oh shit good question hahahahaa	I gave mine to my daughter

What did you do with your wedding album?

Can’t bear to even open it since the divorce

YES,

YOU WILL RISE
FROM THE ASHES,

BUT THE BURNING
COMES FIRST.

FOR THIS PART,
DARLING,

YOU MUST BE BRAVE.

-KALEN DION

I am allowed the space I need.

Rewrite the affirmation

What do you call your kid's other parent?

Write your answer in the box above

Follower Responses (Circle Ones You Connect With)

Devil reencarnated	asshole in my thoughts and his name when i have to talk with him	the sperm donor
Douche Bag (DB for short)	daughter's dad in her presence	the kid's mom
my ex husband	former partner	their other parent
Father of my children	father of my kids when they are around (different things when they're not)	my co-parent

What do you call your kid's other parent?

Wasband

YOUR KIDS DID NOT CAUSE YOUR DIVORCE.

SO STOP INVOLVING THEM IN IT.

-ANTHONY BOMPIANI

@anthonybompiani

I am unstoppable now

Rewrite the affirmation

What's a text you'd like to send to your ex, but won't?

Everyone sees through your BS	Can we talk? (I did it)	You are not worthy as a dad
Once a cheater always a cheater-- wait for it - he aint gonna be faithful to you!	Me vs You: 0	Go fuck yourself. I do not owe you anything. And give me that picture frame my gpa made!
Sorry you lost your job, but karma is a bitch...	So many. I send them to my therapist instead	You are a narcissist sociopath whose abusive process has spent all of my money we had
Leave me alone, while you have the kids it's your turn to figure it out	You think you are so evolved but you are the biggest fucking mess I've ever met	I'm not even sure I can/should type it here.

What's a text you'd like to send to your ex, but won't?

How long did you know, and why didn’t you tell me earlier??

Nobody:

Apple Photos: Look at this picture of you + a person that gave you trauma.

@JalenAndFriends

WRITE A MESSAGE TO YOUR EX (AND DON'T SEND IT)

JUST BECAUSE IT COULD HAVE BEEN DIFFERENT, DOESN'T MEAN IT WOULD HAVE BEEN.

STOP BLAMING YOURSELF FOR WHY IT ENDED OR DIDN'T WORK.

IT TAKES TWO PEOPLE TO MAKE A RELATIONSHIP HAPPEN.

-SABRINA ZOHAR
@do.the.work.podcast

I'm perfect as I am

Rewrite the affirmation

What's 1 thing you learned you're not responsible for in divorce?

I'm not responsible for raising my ex.	My ex partner's narrative of me	His actions
Making sure my side is told... who cares	The tone in which a text message is read.	what they think of me as a partner
I am not responsible for making everyone feel ok cuz a lot of this will feel awful and that is ok	Maintaining relationships with people who weren't supportive	Convincing other people why I wanted/needed a divorce
What people 'think' happened.	The happiness or reactions of other	Cleaning up other people's messes.

What's 1 thing you learned you're not responsible for in divorce?

What people "think" happened.

LEARN TO BE OKAY WITH PEOPLE NOT KNOWING YOUR SIDE OF THE STORY.

YOU HAVE NOTHING TO PROVE TO ANYONE.

-UNKNOWN

WTF

Everything is happening as it should

Rewrite the affirmation

Has your family supported your ex more than you feel like they should?

Yes!!! It's the worst	Some of them, Yes. Like, where is the loyalty?	No, I think they want to sting him up
I feel my exs family supported me more than him and it makes me sad for him. His mom took it pretty hard	No	I had a case where mom moved in BD and the kids and kicked her own daughter out
No, and his family has actually supported me more but he cheated and left...so...	My ex's family supports me more than they do him. They know he's a covert abuser	No, they want to preserve their relationship with their grandkids
Yes... they can't get over our "perfect" relationship	No. But my ex FIL has a better relationship with me than my ex.	No, they celebrated it when I filed for divorce and said "we never liked him anyways"

Has your family supported your ex more than you feel like they should?

Yes he had an affair, 3yrs later he is dating her again and my parents are still his BFF!

I'm kinda like the total package that got fucked up thru shipping and handling.

-Unknown

"I DON'T THINK YOU HAVE TO HAVE SOMEONE WITH YOU ALL THE TIME.

I REALLY DO ENJOY MY WORK, MY KIDS, MY CREATIVE SELF, THAT SOMETIMES — I GOT STIFLED.

LIKE IN RELATIONSHIPS, IT'S HARD TO BE AS CREATIVE AS I CAN BECAUSE I WEAR MY HEART ON MY SLEEVE, SO I REALLY ENJOY [BEING SINGLE]."

-KELLY CLARKSON
@kellyclarkson

I am enough

Rewrite the affirmation

Have you lost your relationship with your ex in-laws? Are you ok/hurt by it?

Write your answer in the box above

Follower Responses (Circle Ones You Connect With)

Your in laws are going to chosse their own child, no matter how wrong they were	I really miss my mother and sisters in law	I didn't actually. We keep in touch because of my son. My son is happy, I am happy too.
Hell. I lost my relationship with my own mother.. and aunt and half my family. F the inlaws.	Yep! Totally ok with it. Blood is thicker than water; accept that & it will help!	Yup. They took his side, knowing his abusive ways & the don't reach out to our kids
Yes, ok with it	My relationship is better now. He told them lies about me.	Relieved!!
It's brutal. Hosted thanksgiving for 23 for 15 years- this year will just be me and kids	Definitely lost the relationship after MIL tried to blame me for him cheating	I have and I am 1,000% okay with it. They were just as Toxic as him

Have you lost your relationship with your ex in-laws? Are you ok/hurt by it?

My relationship is better now. He told them lies about me.

What's something you'd like to say to your mother-in-law (but won't)

What's something you'd like to say to your father-in-law (but won't)

"THE BRICK HOUSES THAT CAN'T BE BLOWN DOWN ARE BUILT WITH POSITIVE SELF-TALK, SELF-VALIDATION, AND LETTING GO OF THE NEED TO BE UNDERSTOOD.

-JAY SKIBBENS
@jayskibbens

IT WILL NEVER BE PERFECT.

DO YOUR BEST AND MAKE IT FUCKING WORK.

-DENISE ALEXANDRA
@abeautifulmindsetcoaching

I am worth the effort

Rewrite the affirmation

How have your friendships changed after divorce?

Write your answer in the box above

Follower Responses (Circle Ones You Connect With)

I'm trying to figure out how to make friends because I put him and the kids first!	I lost my best friends. Never thought that would happen	Yes, its fine. I wished them good luck and said goodbye.
They've become stronger and deeper. Everyone says I'm so proud of you. It's about time.	I found out who really cares for me and who enables my ex	My true people have really shown up and everyone else I'm find letting go of
I lost my best friend of years thru my divorce	I acknowledge that I could be the one reaching out	Making a comeback!!!
So much stronger! All my friends HATED my ex!	I feel bad when they don't reach out to do things when I don't have my kids.	Found my worth & out matured a few so a natural distance has happened.

How have your friendships changed after divorce?

So many are afraid to even talk to me about it, like it's contagious or something.

Shoutout to my best friend for giving me the best advice even though I don't listen.

**I love you
and I'm sorry.**

Don't give up.

-Unknown

Who's a friend who supported you during your divorce?

Write them a short text to share what that meant to you

CHECK ON FRIENDS GOING THROUGH A DIVORCE.

MAKE SURE THEY'RE NOT WAKING UP ALONE DURING THE HOLIDAYS.

THEY WILL NOT CALL YOU FIRST.

NO MATTER HOW AMICABLE THE SPLIT IS, THEY DON'T WANT TO BOTHER YOUR FAMILY CELEBRATION.

-JULIE BURTON
@ksujulie

WTF

I will be happy despite everything

Rewrite the affirmation

Did you lose friends who chose sides in your divorce?

Yes, and it being years later was completely shocking	**This part really sucks but you do get to know who your real friends are.**	**Yes. Didn't realize they were really just her friends, though**
Unfriended and blocked on social media because they believed his side of the story.	**I chose to remove them. But yes. And I'm better for it. I chose people who chose me.**	**Only ones that found out about divorce thru gossip and they didn't reach out!**
Absolutely- sided with cheating husband.	**Nope. In fact, my in laws took my side over her.**	**Yes, but gained so many more along the way and build stronger ones too.**
Yes. Mostly because I dont trust them- they support the abuser disguised as a victim	**Sure did. Lost my family (parents, siblings, aunt, uncle, cousin) too. They picked him**	**I chose to let go of friends who were friends of x to keep things as uncomplicated as possible**

Did you lose friends who chose sides in your divorce?

Yeah, they showed their true colors. Surprised me.

Who's a friend who disappointed you during your divorce?

Write them a short text to share how that affected you

WHEN YOU CHOOSE PEACE, IT COMES WITH A LOT OF GOODBYES.

-UNKNOWN

Things I stopped doing after my divorce:

- **Settling**
- **Being a people pleaser**
- **Making space for anyone who doesn't make space for me**
- **Trying to convince people to be part of my life if they don't make a consistent effort on their own**
- **Dealing with general bullshittery from others**

-RACHEL SOBEL
@whineandcheezits

I am deserving of love

Rewrite the affirmation

Did you unfriend a lot of your ex's friends?

He doesn't have a single friend (should have been a scorching red flag) so, nope.	Nah. Just his family	Nope. The marital challenges are not for public consumption.
They sure showed where their allegiances lied	Hell yea	Nope. Wanted to expose his probably lying and show what he was missing out on
Yes.	All of them	Noo, I even bought them a beer and popcorn
On FB. I unfriended some of his friends. On insta, I unfriended him and all of his friends/family	Yes. Friends and her side of the family.	Yep and had a thing with one of them for a year or so after

Did you unfriend a lot of your ex's friends?

**Yup Blocked some too.
It was so empowering.
Like, "bye bitch"**

**I DON'T HOLD GRUDGES...
WE'RE GOOD.**

**YOU MAY NOT HEAR
FROM ME AGAIN...
BUT WE'RE GOOD.**

-UNKNOWN

Don't mistake my kindness for weakness

Rewrite the affirmation

What's the hardest part about dating after divorce?

Finding the motivation to have any desire to date

Yes schedules!! and the guilt of taking away when schedules don't match up!

It feels so overwhelming

trying to talk to someone who doesn't already know everything about me, and being interesting

Finding someone that gets it and single parenting but heart's still healing making it tough.

The schedule/ finding help to watch kids

I don't want someone else's kids more than I've mine.

Working on yourself but also wanting the company of others

I have zero dating experience (we had been together since HS).

Dating men who haven't done the work on themselves

100% parenting calendar. Inconsistent schedule with my ex due to work travel!

Figuring out if a new potential partner truly is ready for the shit show

What's the hardest part about dating after divorce?

Trusting my self again to pick a good partner

**If you love someone,
set them free.**

**If they come back,
it means nobody
liked them.**

Set them free again.

-UNKNOWN

"YOU'RE NOT GOING TO KNOW WHAT YOU ARE GOING TO FEEL IN THE FUTURE."

-KARA FRANCIS
@karafranciscoaching

Dating apps "wrapped" would be like:

- **you swiped left 100,000x**
- **you swiped right 25x**
- **you shut the app in disgust a lot**
- **you took 800 screenshots of comically bad profiles**
- **you saw 50,000 unsolicited fish pics**
- **you successfully eliminated every single man in a 90-mile radius**

-SARA K. RUNNELS
@omgskr

WTF

LIFE DOESN'T GIVE YOU THE PEOPLE YOU WANT,

IT GIVES YOU THE PEOPLE YOU NEED.

TO HELP YOU,
TO HURT YOU,
TO LOVE YOU,
TO LEAVE YOU,

AND TO MAKE YOU INTO THE PERSON YOU WERE MEANT TO BE.

-MARK GROVES
@createthelove

Boundaries are for me, not them

Rewrite the affirmation

What's a relationship truth you learned from your divorce?

Healing from trauma doesn't mean you're damaged goods	You don't have to beg	Accepting that I don't have to fight to keep someone in love with me, hard to let go though
it's me. hi. I'm the problem it's me.	You don't have to prove yourself worthy of someone's love	You don't have to prove yourself worthy" should be a bumper sticker
Bare minimum isn't actually effort	Actions over words	Believe actions not words. The bare minimum is not effort.
Choosing people that CHOOSE YOU	People will show you what they feel about you.	All. Of. It.

What's a relationship truth you learned from your divorce?

Just because they didn't see your value doesn't mean you're not valuable

**WHEN YOU SAY YES
WHEN YOU MEAN NO,**

**YOU TRADE FEELING
GUILTY IN THE PRESENT
FOR FEELING RESENTFUL
IN THE FUTURE.**

-AMY CHAN
@missamychan

We're not single cause we can't find anyone.

We're single because everytime we find someone, they show us why we're better off single.

-Unknown

“I DO BELIEVE IN LOVE STILL,

BUT I ALSO BELIEVE IT BEGINS WITH REALLY DIGGING DEEP AND LEARNING HOW TO LOVE YOURSELF.”

-JENNA DEWAN
@jennadewan

It's ok to feel lost sometimes

Rewrite the affirmation

5 THINGS I'D TELL MY KID ABOUT RELATIONSHIPS

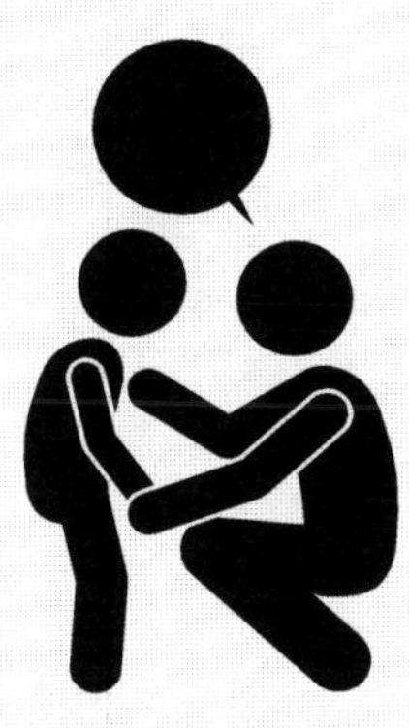

@WTFdivorce

1) A REAL LOVE IS SLOW.

IF THEY SEEM 'OBSESSED' FROM THE START THEY HAVE PUT YOU ON A PEDESTAL THAT WILL BE IMPOSSIBLE TO MAINTAIN.

2) MARRIAGE ISN'T THE GOAL.

THE GOAL IS TO FIND SOMEONE YOU ARE EXCITED ABOUT GOING TO THE GROCERY STORE WITH 5 YEARS LATER AS YOU ARE FOR YOUR FIRST DATE.

3) PEOPLE ARE GOING TO CHANGE.

YOU ARE GOING TO CHANGE.

DON'T FAULT YOU OR YOUR PARTNER.

GO INTO THE RELATIONSHIP KNOWING IT'S SOMEONE YOU ARE EXCITED TO GROW WITH.

4) INTIMACY IS PHYSICAL AND EMOTIONAL.

(SORRY KIDS), BUT SEX IS IMPORTANT; BOTH PARTIES SHOULD BE INVESTED IN THE ENJOYMENT OF THE OTHER.

THE MORE EMOTIONAL SUPPORT YOU CONSISTENTLY PROVIDE WILL TRANSLATE DIRECTLY TO DESIRE.

5) YOU HAVE PERMISSION TO END ANY RELATIONSHIP THAT DOESN'T SERVE YOU.

YOU ARE NEVER STUCK.

UNDERSTANDING WHEN YOU AREN'T COMPATIBLE OR HAPPY IS A SKILL.

PRACTICE IT WHILE YOU ARE YOUNG.

What's 1 thing you want your kids to learn about relationships?

"I'M GRATEFUL FOR ALL THAT HAS COME AND THANKFUL FOR ALL THAT HAS LEFT.

WHATEVER HAD TO GO WAS NOT MINE."

@wetheurban

I am modeling for my kids

Rewrite the affirmation

What's 1 thing you're going to work on post-divorce?

Become not finacially dependent on him	pulling out	channeling the anger into positivity. letting that sh*t go.
stop procrastinating, making excuses, live the life i've always wanted	knowing who i am	see people for who they show me that are the first time!
getting the past out of my head, letting go of resentment	forgiving myself	managing my emotions without needing to dump them on someone else
not reacting... taking time to respond.	finding happiness within myself and not relying on another person to do that for me.	over-functioning and being clear about what i need.

What's 1 thing you're going to work on post-divorce?

not worrying so much about their feelings, and stop ignoring my own

BE PATIENT WHEN BECOMING SOMEONE YOU HAVEN'T BEEN BEFORE

-TANYA MARKUL
@tanyamarkul

I'm at a point in my life where I don't even know the point I'm at,

but I'm at a point.

-Unknown

TRY AND GIVE YOURSELF SOME EXTRA SPACE, TIME, AND GRACE THIS SEASON.

IT HAS BEEN A HARD YEAR.

-ERIN SCHADEN
@erineschaden

WTF

I am strong

Rewrite the affirmation

Describe your dream vacation

AZ hippie spa stay + hiking + outings at local artsy shops and speakeasles	sun, run book, nap
A beach, cocktails and lots of sunsets	Mountains, trees, frozen pond, snow, skates
A virtual reality where i can kill my ex and not go to jail	A private island oasis
White lotus location and funding - 10 days completely disconnecting	Planning my first solo trip. a little scary after 20 years of marriage.

Describe your dream vacation

me doing my thing, not on anyone else's schedule, not having to make sure someone else is happy

**ONE DAY YOU'RE GOING
TO LOOK BACK
ON THIS TIME**

**WHERE YOU THOUGHT ALL
OF YOUR BEST DAYS HAD
ALREADY HAPPENED,**

**AND WISH THAT YOU
KNEW HOW MANY BETTER
ONES WERE AHEAD.**

-UNKNOWN

I'm ok with my divorce

Rewrite the affirmation

REAL JOURNAL EXCERPTS

-ANONYMOUS

I don't know what kind of cruel trick the universe is playing on me, or what the life wisdom God is trying to teach me, but my heart is hurting from all of the lies and cheating.

But I fought, and I fought hard. For my children, my husband, my family. We're all going to be okay in the end, I just wish it didn't have to turn out like this.

with all of my heart and tried so
incredibly hard to push through and keep/
save our marriage. It just wasn't enough.
I don't know what cruel trick the
universe is playing on me or what
life wisdom God is trying to teach me,
but my heart is hurting from all of
the lies and cheating. But I fought,
and I fought hard. For my children,
my husband, my family. We're all going
to be okay in the end, I just wish
it didn't have to turn out like this.
Now I have to re-invent myself.
And I don't know where to begin.
My self-confidence is shot, but slowly
coming back, and I have no idea
who I am or who I'm supposed to
be. I watched some inspirational clip
about Tiffany Haddish yesterday. She
said to write down your goals, work

REAL JOURNAL EXCERPTS

-ANONYMOUS

I don't understand how he gets to have it so easy. Why?

When will someone love me? I almost texted him today. I guess that's how it is with him. He will avoid forever and if he never has to have the conversations, then it never happened.

I hate this. I can't wait until I'm living a life without him. Completely. I don't want to hurt anymore. I don't want to love him anymore. I just want our kids to be happy, and me to be happy. I don't want to feel like that's selfish. I'm so tired of crying. When will I get a GOD DAMN BREAK?!

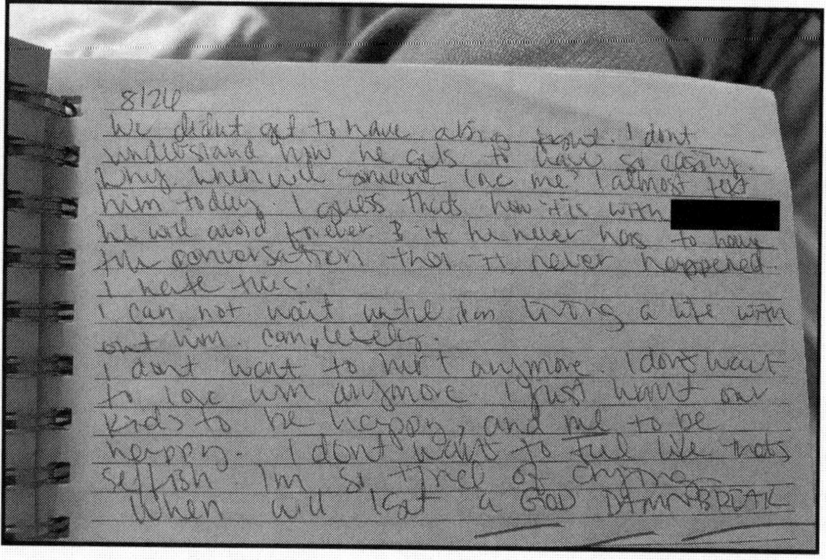

8/24
We didnt get to have a big [illegible]. I dont
understand how he gets to have so easy.
Why. When will someone love me? I almost text
him today. I guess thats how it is with [redacted]
he will avoid forever & if he never has to have
the conversation then it never happened.
I hate this.
I can not wait until I'm living a life with
out him. completely.
I dont want to hurt anymore. I dont want
to love him anymore. I just want our
kids to be happy, and me to be
happy. I dont want to feel like thats
selfish. I'm so tired of crying.
When will I get a GOD DAMN BREAK

REAL JOURNAL EXCERPTS

-ANONYMOUS

Okay, let's start again.

Currently I'm a divorced mom of two. Not at all what I wanted, but I have to accept it and work through it. I have a lot of feelings of inadequacy, embarrassment, anger, and sadness.

...maybe it's that I don't really feel like I have what it takes to be lovable.

But my goal by the end is to love myself, be sincerely charming and gorgeous and have a strong foundation of kindness, confidence, and poise.

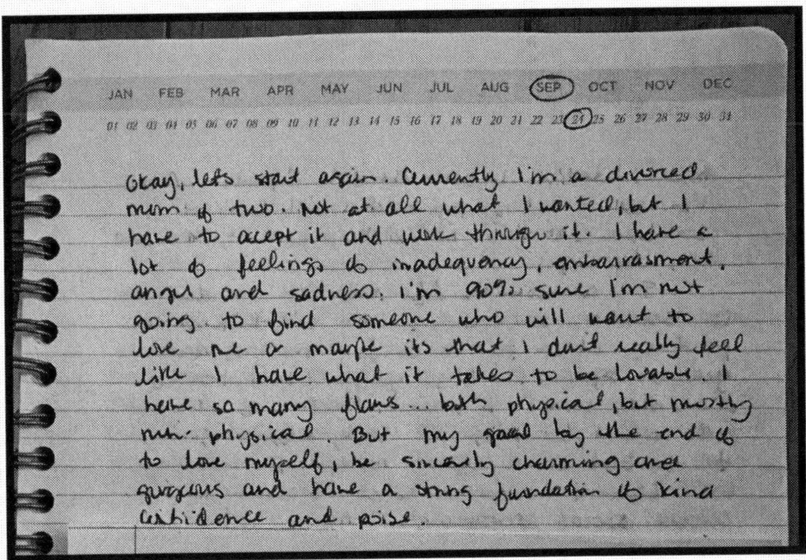

JAN FEB MAR APR MAY JUN JUL AUG SEP OCT NOV DEC

01 02 03 04 05 06 07 08 09 10 11 12 13 14 15 16 17 18 19 20 21 22 23 24 25 26 27 28 29 30 31

Okay, lets start again. Currently I'm a divorced
mom of two. not at all what I wanted, but I
have to accept it and work through it. I have a
lot of feelings of inadequacy, embarrassment,
anger and sadness. I'm 90% sure I'm not
going to find someone who will want to
love me or maybe its that I don't really feel
like I have what it takes to be lovable. I
have so many flaws... both physical, but mostly
non-physical. But my goal by the end is
to love myself, be sincerely charming and
gorgeous and have a strong foundation of kind
confidence and poise.

REAL JOURNAL EXCERPTS

-ANONYMOUS

Remain strong at all costs.

Keep yourself together and "happy".
Don't let them see the truth.
The truth is, I had strayed so far from my own essence.
I reached a point where I could barely feel her anymore.

When I ultimately journeyed through my own 'rock bottom', I experienced the most expansive transformation of my life. I learned that you can derive more strength from rock bottom status than just about anywhere. It can bee one of the most raw and beautiful states of consciousness. If we let it be.

View From The Bottom

Rock Bottom. A term I had heard many times and yet had a very modest view of. I considered it to be a blanket term for a person, namely from substance abuse or something of that nature, that just simply couldn't go on any further in that state of being. At that point, they are forced to stop. A word that generated fear in me. I assumed it meant weakness. Or end of life. Trying to avoid that state seemed like the goal all humans were trying to achieve. It felt like the mission of my lifetime. Remain strong at all costs. Keep yourself together and "happy". Don't let them see the truth. The truth is, I had strayed so far from my own essence. I reached a point where I could barely feel her anymore. When I ultimately journeyed through my own Rock Bottom, I experienced the most expansive transformation of my lifetime. I learned that you can derive more strength from rock bottom status than just about anywhere. It can be one of the most raw and beautiful states of consciousness. If we let it be.

My new belief is that rock bottom is simply an invitation to ourselves. It is permission to strip away everything and rebirth yourself. We avoid it at all costs because it is an excruciating place to be in. Humans are programmed to run from pain. We distract, we numb and we avoid. Until sometimes, we simply can't. We don't have the energy to fight it away anymore. We make a choice. We choose to put one foot in front of the other. Then we surrender. We fold into the rock bottom status. We don't know how long we will visit there. We trust. We have faith. We realize that no thought or feeling we have will impact the flow of life. Life will happen as it meant to. Every single time. We lean into the pain, buckle up and breathe.

REAL JOURNAL EXCERPTS

-ANONYMOUS

████ and I are getting a divorce.

After a year and a half in limbo (at least for me), he asked me again for the 3rd time this year (that's 4 total if we're keeping track) along with the disclosure that he had strong feelings and was sleeping with a college classmate.

If your husband cheats on you twice and falls in love while doing so, and asks you for a divorce 4 times, and buys a condo on his own, and moves out, I guess it's time to throw in the towel.

One thing I'm sure of: I fought.

thought into my observations. And so, here we are.
████ and I are getting a divorce. After a year and a half in limbo (at least for me), he asked me again for the 3rd time this year (thats 4 total if were keeping track) along with the disclosure that he had strong feelings and was sleeping with a college classmate ████ If your husband cheats on you twice and falls in love while doing so and asks you for a divorce 4 times and buys a condo on his own and moves out, I guess its time to throw in the towel. One thing I'm sure of: I fought

I am capable of loving again

Rewrite the affirmation

CLOSING THOUGHTS

Whew. Who ever said you were afraid of commitment? You made it.

Our most successful relationship has been with all of you. While we have related to, laughed at, and been humbled by all the comments, DMs and story replies over the past 2 years; this journal is entirely yours to do with as you please.

Revisit it as you move forward in your journey, hide it in your closet, light it on fire, or hang your favorite entries on the fridge.

Most importantly though; take pride in the fact that you are doing the hard things.

Congratulations on facing the tough stuff and thank you for being a part of this community.

ONE LAST THING

Before you go....for **3 FREE bonus** WTF prompts and a sneak peek at the next edition, go to:

www.WTFdivorce.com/journal

Just pop in your email and we'll send it over.

***

If you find this book helpful, **please leave a quick review** on Amazon, and tell your friends about it.

This helps it find its way to those who need it, and it would really mean a lot to us.

Thank you.
-Rob

MORE WTF DIVORCE

Podcasts: If you like listening to podcasts and want to hear more, check out our 5-star rated shows:

- WTF Divorce
- Co-Parenting Help
- Ask A Divorce Lawyer
- I Think I Want A Divorce

Videos: Check our our YouTube (search WTF divorce)

Courses: If you'd like help with co-parent communication, check out our video course at: www.wtfdivorce.com

Instagram: If you like quick tips, inspiring quotes, and hilarious memes, join 117,000 followers on our Instagram @WTFdivorce

***

And last, thank you again. Please be one of those givers and **share this with other friends dealing with divorce by leaving a review.**

It would mean the world to us.

ABOUT THE AUTHORS

Rob Roseman is a divorced dad to 3 kids, former Las Vegas poker pro, author of the 5-star rated book, Dad the Best I Can, and the founder of WTF Divorce. In his (rare) spare time, he enjoys going to see stand-up comedy, laughing with old friends, and watching the Miami Heat. Born and raised in Miami, FL, Rob currently lives in Roswell, GA.

Kristy Tiesing is a divorced mom to 2 kids, former high school teacher, and freelance online business owner. When she is not busy with responsibilities of single parenting or client work, you can find her in the gym, enjoying a good book, or working on the farm in mid-Missouri where she currently lives.

INDEX

S.C. Lourie	7	Jacquelyn Tenaglia	95
Cindy Stibbard	24	Anthony Bompiani	108
Alessandra Martinet	25, 92	Jay Skibbens	129
Michelle Dempsey	34	Denise Alexandra	130
Barbara Mezei	36	Julie Burton	136
Joél Leon	39	Rachel Sobel	143
Kristy Tiesing	44,192	Kara Francis	152
Andrea Rappaport	60	Sara K. Runnels	153
Tracy Moore-Grant	61	Mark Groves	155
Meagan Norris	65	Amy Chan	159
Sadie Marie	66	Tanya Markul	174
Heidi Brocke	68	Erin Schaden	176
Sabrina Zohar	86,114	Rob Roseman	192
Bradley Richardson	88		

Made in the USA
Middletown, DE
19 July 2024